Lynda Aoudia

Imaging breast anatomy

AF301749

Lynda Aoudia

Imaging breast anatomy

ScienciaScripts

Imprint

Any brand names and product names mentioned in this book are subject to trademark, brand or patent protection and are trademarks or registered trademarks of their respective holders. The use of brand names, product names, common names, trade names, product descriptions etc. even without a particular marking in this work is in no way to be construed to mean that such names may be regarded as unrestricted in respect of trademark and brand protection legislation and could thus be used by anyone.

Cover image: www.ingimage.com

This book is a translation from the original published under ISBN 978-620-6-71379-1.

Publisher:
Sciencia Scripts
is a trademark of
Dodo Books Indian Ocean Ltd. and OmniScriptum S.R.L publishing group

120 High Road, East Finchley, London, N2 9ED, United Kingdom
Str. Armeneasca 28/1, office 1, Chisinau MD-2012, Republic of Moldova, Europe
Printed at: see last page
ISBN: 978-620-7-67416-9

Copyright © Lynda Aoudia
Copyright © 2024 Dodo Books Indian Ocean Ltd. and OmniScriptum S.R.L publishing group

Imaging breast anatomy

Lynda AOUDIA

Foreword

Breast cancer is the most common cancer in women worldwide. Breast imaging (mammography, ultrasound and MRI) is the fundamental means of exploring the mammary gland. Good correlation of imaging data with anatomical, histological and physiological data enables a better understanding of the image produced. Mammographic, ultrasound and MRI variations are encountered, generally due to constitutional factors, but also to individual physiological variations and exogenous factors. A good knowledge of normal breast anatomy enables better detection of breast anomalies.

Prof. Lynda AOUDIA

Table of contents

Introduction

The challenge in interpreting breast imaging (mammography, ultrasound) is to detect abnormal images within a glandular structure that is unique to each individual, and for which there is no reference standard. Basic anatomical imaging varies for different parts of the gland, depending on the period of the cycle and the different stages of life. Mammography, ultrasound and MRI each provide their own specific information, with variable performance depending on the glandular structure. For mammography, it is essential to have previous documents showing the patient's basic mapping, so that they can be compared with the examination performed. Ultrasound, on the other hand, does not allow this comparative study. Knowledge of embryonic data is fundamental to understanding certain developmental anomalies, as well as certain anatomical, histological and physiological data to better detect the abnormal image. The construction of the gland is genetically determined, but the glandular tissue will undergo individual variations, depending on endogenous factors such as age and the period of the menstrual cycle, and also on exogenous factors, such as changes in weight and hormone treatment. The image produced is the result of the many elements that make up the mammary gland.

Breast anatomy

1. Embryological basis

The breasts are of ectodermal origin. They develop as early as 5^e weeks gestation from the mammary crest, extending from the root of the upper limbs, along the ventral surface of the embryo, to the root of the lower limbs (fig. 1). Two symmetrical mammary buds appear at the level of this crest, in a pectoral position. These buds form the areola-mammary plate (AMP), then invaginate into the underlying mesoderm to form the milk ducts (fig. 1). These in turn evolve to form glandular units or lobes [1].

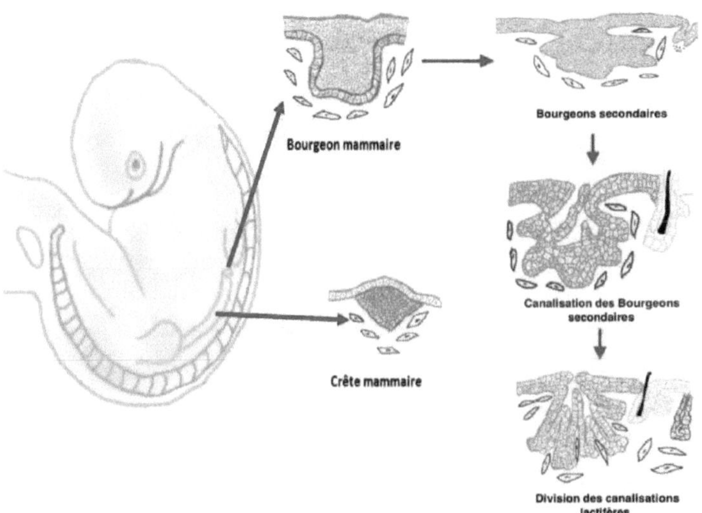

Fig. 1: Embryogenesis of the mammary gland.

2. Anatomical basis [2-9]

2.1. Anatomy of the mammary gland

The mammary gland lies in front of the chest wall, between the clavicle and the 6ᵉ or 8ᵉ rib, and laterally, it extends from the sternum to the middle axillary line.

2.1.1. The skin covering

The skin covering of the breast is not homogeneous, and three concentric zones are described (fig. 2):

- Skin: smooth, supple.

- Areola: pigmented, circular, 35 to 50 mm in diameter.

- The nipple: located in the center of the areola.

2.1.2. Glandular tissue

It is organized into around twenty lobes. Each lobe is made up of 20 to 40 lobules, each with an excretory duct or galactophore duct, into which the secondary ducts drain, each leading to a ducto-lobular terminal unit (DLTU), consisting of a terminal duct, collecting several acini (fig. 3).

The milk ducts converge towards the nipple, widening to form the lactiferous sinuses, then narrowing and opening into the nipple pores.

2.1.3. Connective tissue

Two types of connective tissue are described:

- Interlobar connective tissue, surrounding the mammary lobules and lobes, extends to the anterior surface of the gland, forming Cooper's ligaments that are attached to the skin by Duret's ridges (fig. 2).

- The intra-lobular connective tissue surrounding the inner ducts of each lobule is called pallial tissue (fig. 3).

2.1.4. Adipose tissue

Adhered to glandular tissue, the quantity of adipose tissue is primarily responsible for breast size.

Two fatty layers can be distinguished (fig. 2):

- The anterior pre-glandular layer does not exist at the level of the nipple-areolar plate. It is partitioned by Cooper's ligaments.
- The posterior, retroglandular layer is bounded by the fascia superficialis.

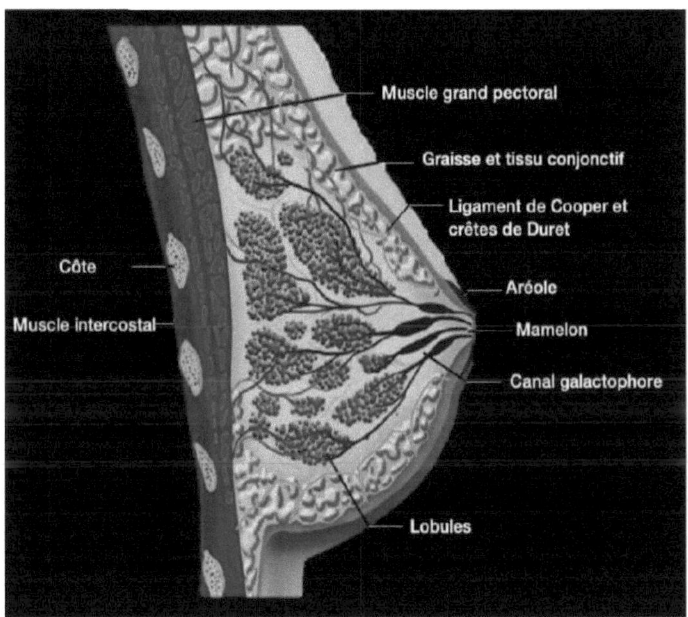

Fig. 2. Anatomical structure of the breast.

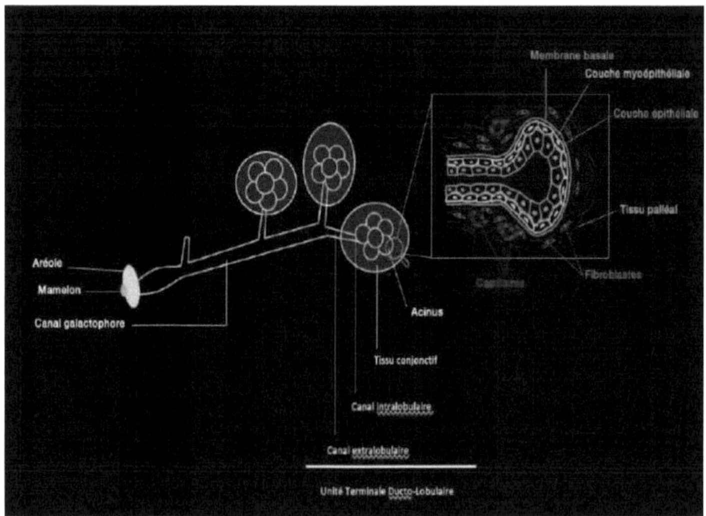

Fig. 3: Schematic representation of the ducto-lobular end unit.

2.2. Vascular anatomy of the breast

The superior-external part of the gland is vascularized by branches of the axillary artery, the central and internal part by perforating branches of the internal mammary artery; the external part of the gland mainly receives branches of the intercostal arteries (fig. 4).

Venous drainage is divided into the superficial venous network, which drains into the superficial veins of neighboring regions, and the deep venous network, which accompanies the arterial network. The deep veins drain into the external mammary veins laterally, the internal mammary vein medially and the intercostal veins posteriorly.

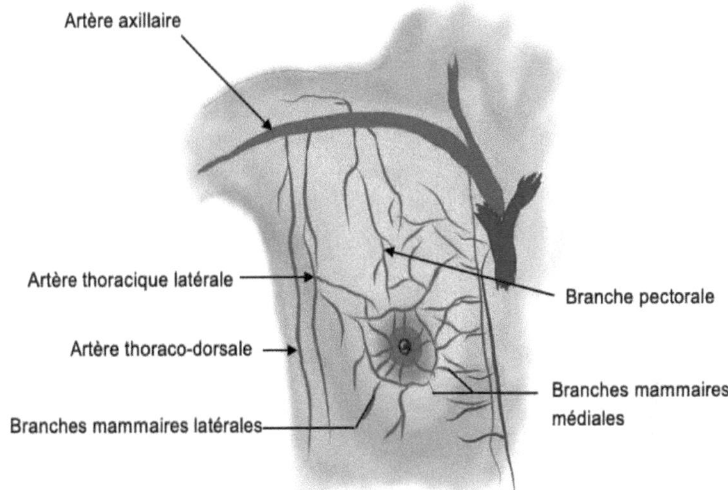

Fig. 4: Vascularization of the breast.

2.3. Breast lymph drainage

Lymphatic drainage takes place from deep within the glandular tissue to peri-areolar lymphatic plexuses. Three-quarters of drainage is from lateral and medial trunks, from the areola to the armpit, the remainder from the internal mammary chain. Anastomoses exist with the contralateral breast [10].

The nodes are divided into three levels, known as Berg's levels, according to their position in relation to the pectoralis minor muscle (fig. 5) [11] :

- Level I (lower axilla): the lymph nodes are located below the pectoralis minor muscle;

- level II (middle axillary stage): the lymph nodes are located behind the pectoralis minor muscle;

- level III (upper axilla): lymph nodes are located above the pectoralis minor muscle.

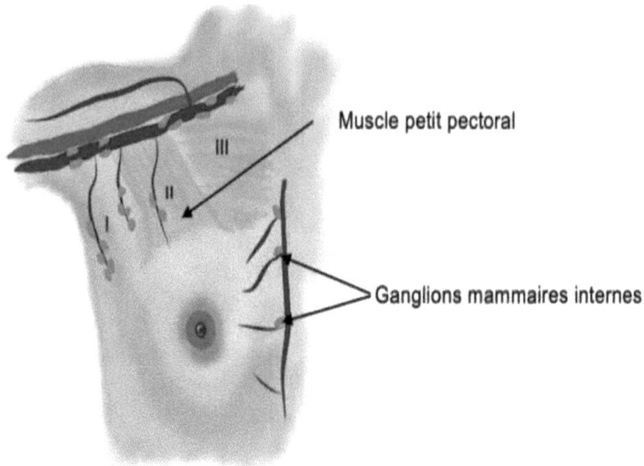

Fig. 5. Berg's three levels of lymph nodes and internal mammary nodes.

2.4 Innervation

Sensory innervation of the breast comes from lateral and anterior cutaneous perforating branches of the 2eme to 7eme intercostal nerves. The lower branches of the superficial cervical plexus also contribute to innervation of the upper part of the breast.

3. Physiological basis

The architecture of the mammary gland evolves throughout life, depending on age and stage of reproductive life [12, 13], under the influence of sex hormones of ovarian origin (estrogen and progesterone) and a number of growth factors (fig. 6).

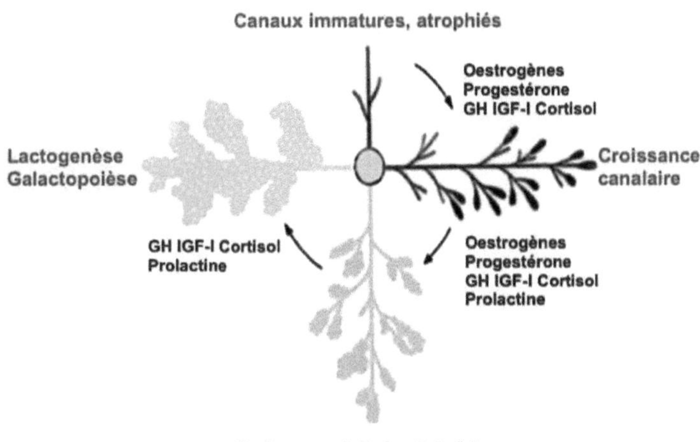

Fig. 6: Schematic representation of mammary gland development [14].

Imaging techniques

1. Mammography

Mammography is the reference radiological examination for screening for breast cancer, the leading cause of death in women.

Mammographic images must be optimized in terms of spatial resolution, contrast and noise. A number of technical criteria need to be taken into account, including high contrast for good visualization of microcalcifications. The radiation spectrum must be broad, to adapt to varying breast densities, and the radiation dose must be minimal, especially in young patients.

1.1. Impact

Positioning the breast is a fundamental step in mammography, and the technique must be beyond reproach. The aim is to radiograph the entire mammary gland, including the deep planes. Positioning is the key to obtaining optimal images, essential for interpretation, and meeting a number of quality criteria [15].

1.1.1. Fundamental impacts

1.1.1.1.Cranio-caudal or frontal incision

The X-ray beam approaches the breast craniocaudally (fig. 7).

The difficulty of the front view lies in the absence of visualization of the deep mammary planes, and it is important to engage as much posterior mammary tissue as possible.

The criteria for successful incidence are (fig. 8):

- The breast is at the center of the image.
- The gland is well spread out.

- The nipple is at its zenith [16].
- No folds or overlaps.

The pectoralis muscle is visible in almost 30% of cases, and its presence on the x-ray allows optimum depth gain [15].

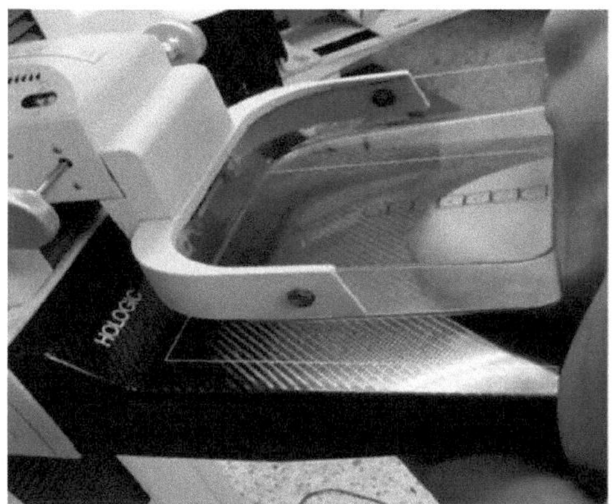

Fig. 7. Front incision.

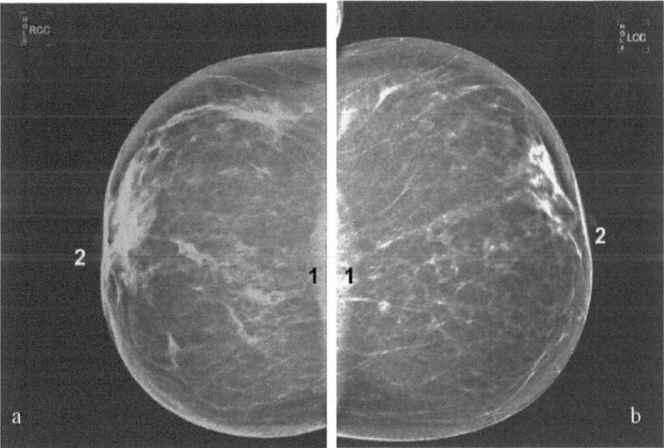

Fig. 8: Quality criteria for frontal incidence. Mammographic images. (a) Right face. (b) Left face. Pectoral muscle (1), nipple at zenith (2).

1.1.1.2.45° external oblique incidence°

This allows the breast to be studied in its long axis, and a maximum amount of breast tissue to be analyzed [17]. The stand is tilted at a strict 45°° to ensure reproducible incidence (fig. 9).

The difficulty with this incidence is to evenly compress the pectoral muscle, the breast and the submammary fold.

The criteria for successful incidence are (fig. 10)

- The pectoral muscle is visible up to halfway up the image [18].
- The nipple is at its zenith, opposite the tip of the pectoral muscle [17].
- Presence of abdominal wall skin fold [16].
- The long axis of the breast tends towards the horizontal.
- Presence of the "open" submammary fold, perfectly clear of the abdominal wall [19].
- No folds or overlaps.

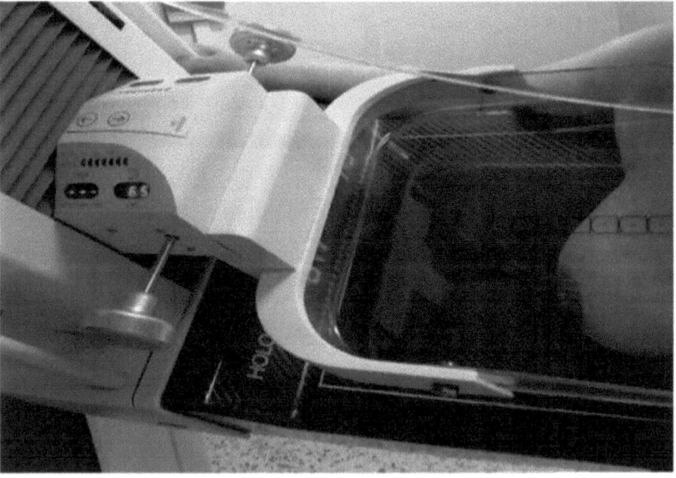

Fig. 9. External oblique incidence.

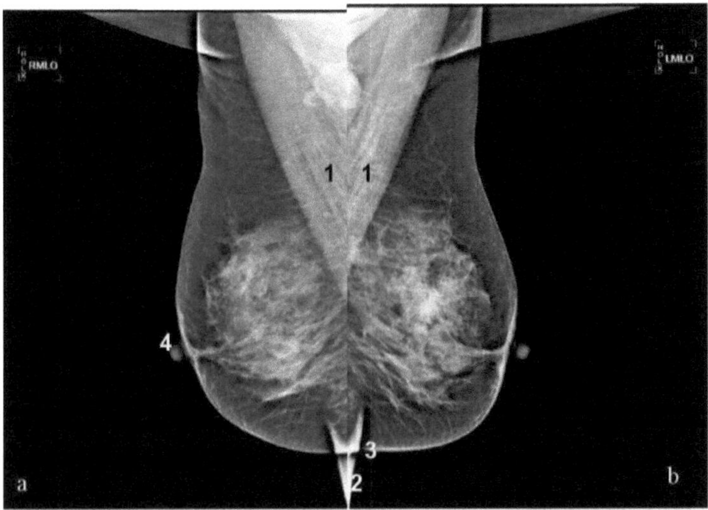

Fig. 10. Quality criteria for external oblique incidence. Mammographic images (a) Right oblique (b) Left oblique. Pectoral muscle (1), abdominal wall skin fold (2), open sub-mammary fold (3), nipple at zenith (4).

1.1.2. Additional impacts

They are always carried out in addition to the fundamental impacts.

1.1.2.1 Profile incidence

It is useful for determining the precise location of a lesion. It can also be used to highlight the sloping nature of microcalcifications.

1.1.2.2. Localized centric view

It can be used to analyze the contours of a nodule or stellate image, or to eliminate a constructed image (fig. 11).

1.1.2.3. Enlarged centered shot

Microcalcifications visible on standard images can be enlarged for detailed analysis (number, appearance, organization, etc.) (fig. 12).

1.1.2.4. Other impacts

Axillary extension, Cleopatra incidence, staggered frontal incidence, tangential cliché, Eklund maneuver [20-23].

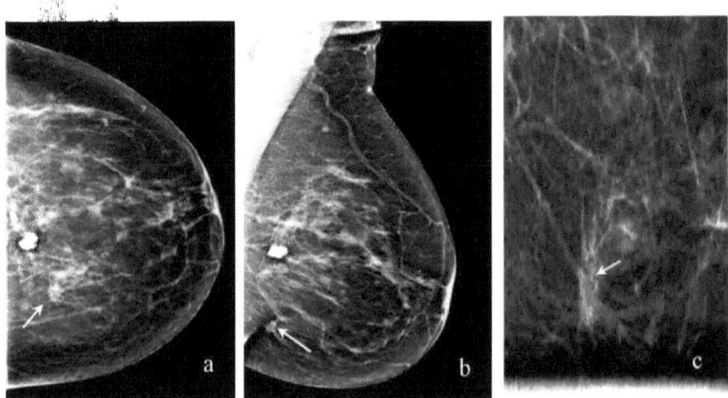

Fig. 11. Localized centric view. (a) Front view. Mass with indistinct contours (arrow). (b) External oblique view. Mass in the sub mammary fold with poorly defined contours (arrow). (c). View centred on the mass. Mass with spiculated contours, BIRADS 5 (arrow).

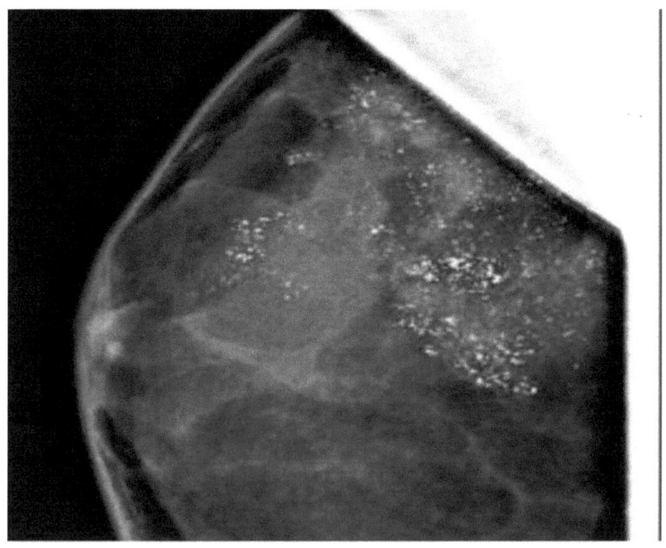

Fig. 12. Enlarged centric view. Magnification of a focus of microcalcifications.

2. Ultrasound

Ultrasound is an accessible, non-irradiating and inexpensive imaging technique. It may be indicated as a complement to mammography, to improve lesion detection, particularly in dense breasts, and to characterize lesions, notably to differentiate solid from cystic lesions, and to take samples [24].

Breast ultrasound is performed with a high-frequency probe, usually between 9 and 15 MHz, for good contrast and spatial resolution [25]. There are several ultrasound modes.

2.1. Mode B

This is the first technique used when performing breast ultrasound. Ultrasound waves are emitted and collected by the probe, at the same frequency, in a single direction. They are combined to create a 2D grayscale image of the breast [26]. This technique enables structures to be differentiated on the basis of the acoustic and mechanical properties of the tissue. This B-mode has a number of weaknesses, including inconsistent optimal resolution and artifacts that can degrade image quality [27] (fig. 13).

2.2. Harmonic mode

It is linked to the non-linear behavior of breast tissue with respect to ultrasound. As the ultrasound wave propagates through breast tissue, it undergoes progressive distortion of the ultrasound pulse shape, creating harmonic frequencies which are multiples of the emission frequency [28-

30]. Once the initial signal has been filtered, the harmonic signal is used for image reconstruction. This technique improves the contrast of ultrasound images, particularly in the case of cysts with "thick contents" or complicated cysts, which show internal echoes in B mode, whereas in harmonic mode they appear anechoic [31] (fig. 13).

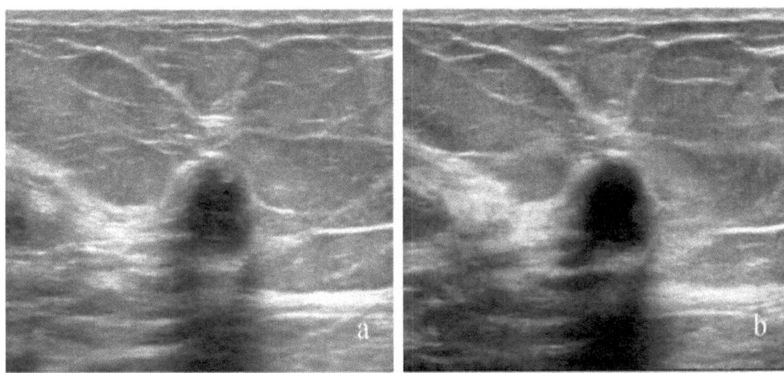

Fig. 13: Harmonic mode (a) B-mode ultrasound. Hypoechoic mass, (b) Harmonic mode ultrasound. Cystic anechogenic mass with thickened wall. Histology. Histology: reworked cyst.

2.3. Composite mode (Compound)

Two types of composite, frequency composite (several different ultrasound emission frequencies are used to reconstruct the final image), and spatial composite (several ultrasound emission angles are used and combined into a single composite image). This technique limits artifacts, improves analysis of lesion contours, better defines the internal echostructure of masses and enables detection of small lesions [32] (fig. 14). It also enables better detection of intra-lesional calcifications [33]. On the other hand, posterior ultrasound changes are attenuated [34].

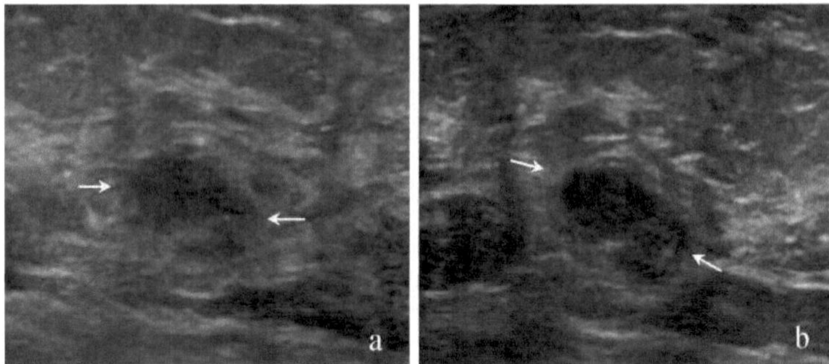

Fig. 14. Composite mode. (a) B-mode ultrasound. Hypoechoic mass with indistinct contours, (b) Composite-mode ultrasound. Hypoechoic, circumscribed mass. Histology: Adenofibroma.

2.4. Doppler mode

It detects tumor angiogenesis. Malignant lesions are generally more vascularized than benign ones, with an abnormal, irregular appearance of the vessels. Detection and spectrum analysis of these vessels require a probe of at least 10 MHz and a rigorous ultrasound technique (adjustment of focus, reduction of overall gain, adaptation of the size of the Doppler box, filtering to the minimum 10 in order to analyze low frequencies, no pressure on the breast to avoid obliteration of small vessels) [35, 36].

Energy Doppler has better sensitivity to slow flows, but is more sensitive to artifacts [34]. Doppler can be used to analyze hypoechoic lesions of a "cystic or solid" nature. The presence of vascularization in an echogenic lesion indicates that the lesion is tissue-based. On the other hand, the absence of vascularization does not rule out the presence of a tissue portion [26] (fig. 15).

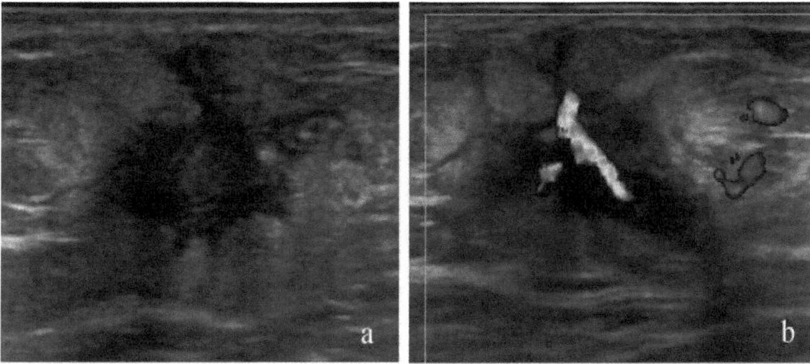

Fig. 15. Doppler mode: (a) B-mode ultrasound. Hypoechoic mass with spiculated contours, (b) Doppler mode ultrasound. Intralesional vascularization.

2.5. Elastography

Elastography is a non-invasive technique used in conjunction with ultrasound to qualitatively, semi-quantitatively or quantitatively assess the deformability of lesions subjected to stress [37, 38]. The image obtained is then translated into an elastogram. This technique was developed to improve the specificity of B-mode breast ultrasound, by adding compressibility and lesion "hardness" to the criteria of echostructure and lesion morphology (fig. 16). Breast elastography uses two distinct modes: free-hand elastography and shear-wave elastography.

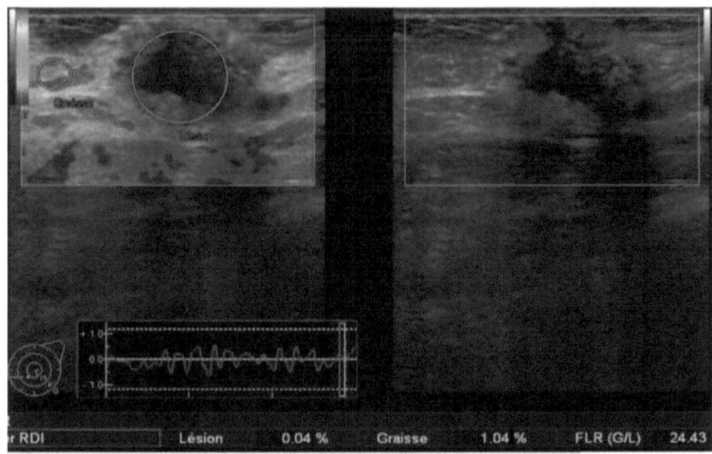

Fig. 16. Elastography. Elastography. Calculation of elasticity ratio in standard deviation.

3. Breast MRI

3.1. Equipment

3.1.1.Magnetic field

Magnetic field strength influences acquisition time and image quality. The higher the magnetic field intensity, the better the image resolution and the shorter the sequence time. Most teams work with magnetic fields of 1.5 tesla (T).

3.1.2. Antennas

Breast MRI must be performed using dedicated breast antennas that follow the shape of the breasts (fig. 17). The use of parallel imaging improves the performance of these antennas, increasing surface coverage, signal uniformity and temporal and spatial resolution [39]. The breasts must be well positioned in the antenna, with the nipple at the zenith, integrating the entire breast into the antenna and avoiding folds (fig. 18).

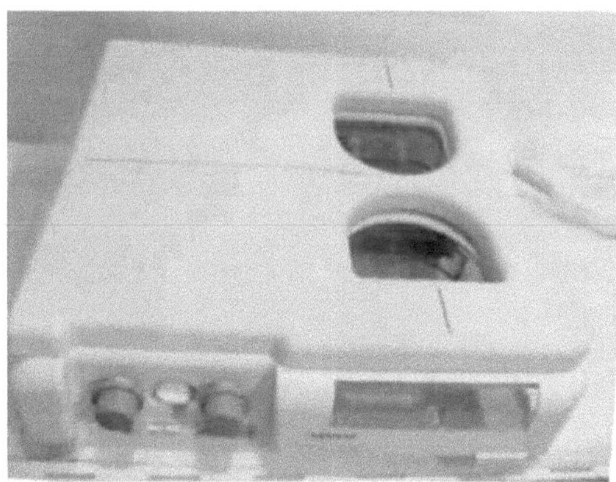

Fig. 17. Antenna breast.

The breast should not be overly compressed. Compression serves to wedge the breasts to prevent their movement in the antenna. Excessive compression of the breast can falsely reduce the size of lesions, thus changing the TNM classification [40]. Compression can also reduce the amplitude of enhancement and alter the enhancement curve (fig. 19).

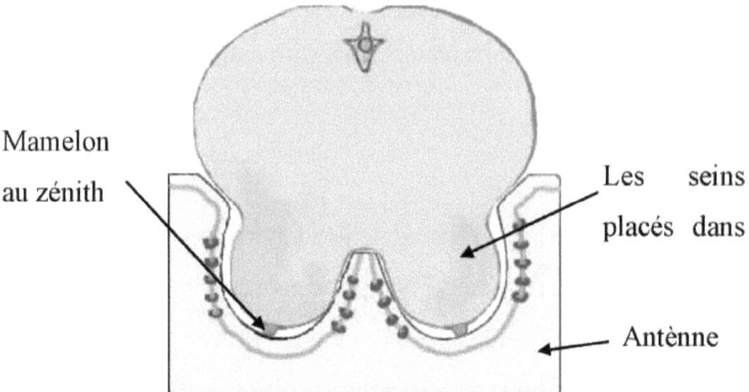

Fig. 18. Position of breasts in the anterior.

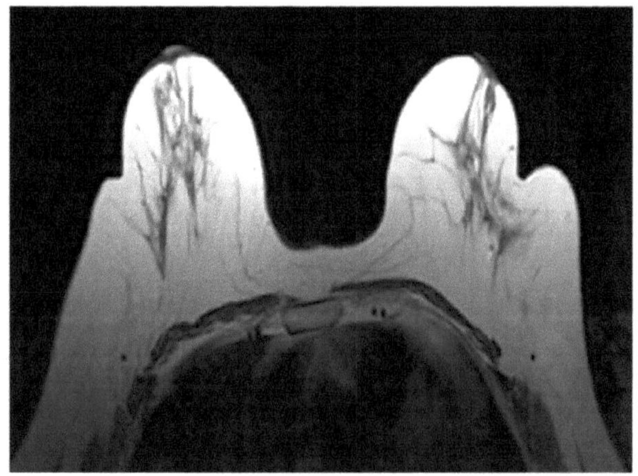

Fig. 19. Compression defect. T2-weighted sequence

3.2. Time of examination

The timing of the examination is essential for the best interpretation of breast MRI. Avoid the second half of the cycle, when physiological glandular enhancement is most marked. It is minimal in the 2nd week of the menstrual cycle in patients with genital activity. Outside this period, non-specific diffuse or focal contrast enhancement may be present, leading to misinterpretation (fig. 20). Glandular enhancement is increased by hormone replacement therapy in post-menopausal women, with up to 50% of women showing non-specific enhancement. In the event of an uninterpretable examination in post-menopausal women, the test should be discontinued for 3 months.

For post-operative MRI, a minimum delay of one month must be observed to limit enhancement secondary to inflammatory phenomena. The optimum time for performing breast MRI is at least six months after the end of treatment [4143].

Percutaneous microbiopsies generally have no impact on the interpretation of contrast-enhanced MRI. However, the topography, date of biopsy and results, if available, should always be mentioned. Oral contraception also has no impact on the use of breast MRI.

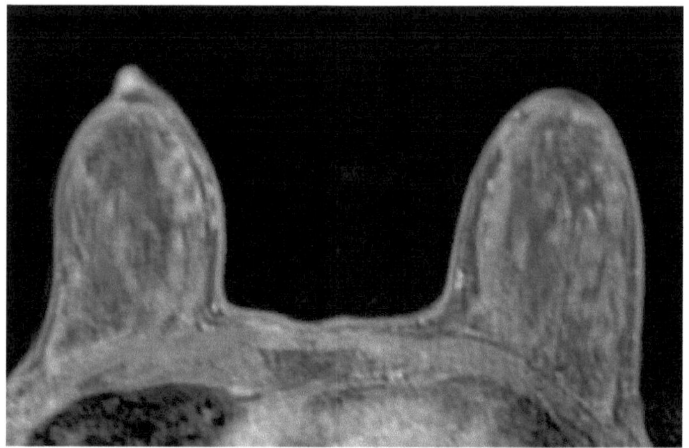

Fig. 20. Physiological glandular enhancement. Subtracted sequence injected.

3.3. Installing the patient

A venous access with long tubing is set up. The patient is then placed in procubitus position, with her arms over her head as comfortably as possible, to ensure the immobility required for the examination. The breasts placed in the antenna must be well supported; if necessary, a foam pad can be used to prevent small breasts from moving in the antenna.

3.4. Injection of contrast media

Breast MRI highlights intratumoral neoangiogenesis through contrast injection, enabling lesions to be detected [44]. The contrast medium used is gadolinium chelate. The injected dose is 0.1 mmol/kg body weight. The injection rate should be 2 to 3 ml per second. Injection of the contrast medium is followed by an injection of 20 ml of saline at the same flow rate, to avoid stagnation of the contrast medium in the tubing.

3.5. Breast MRI protocols

3.5.1. Acquisition plan

Fields of view must be sufficiently wide to allow analysis of both breasts, both nipple-areolar plates (NAPs), the axillary hollows and the chest wall [44, 45].

Acquisition in the axial plane is the most frequently used. This acquisition plane enables dynamic sequences of the breasts to be performed in 1 minute. The advantages of the axial plane are comparative analysis of the whole of both breasts, which facilitates detection of abnormal contrast, and analysis of the PAMs, axillary hollows and chest wall [45]. Cardiorespiratory artifacts degrade acquisition quality. Phase encoding from right to left instead of anteroposterior reduces these artifacts.

Acquisition in the sagittal plane reduces the field of view. This in turn improves image resolution and the quality of fat suppression techniques [44]. Finally, sagittal acquisition also enables better analysis of physiological glandular enhancement, which facilitates anatomical study. Nevertheless, the study of both breasts, including the axillary hollows, requires a large number of slices, which prolongs examination time [45].

Coronal acquisition reduces cardiac artifacts. But this plane is often degraded by respiratory and flow artifacts. This acquisition plane also requires many slices to be able to analyze the entire breast from the chest wall to the PAM [45].

3.5.2. Cutting thickness

Slice thickness must be thin, less than or equal to 3 mm, with pixel and voxel sizes of less than 1 mm. To enable us to carry out multiplanar reconstructions.

3.5.3. Breast MRI sequences

3.5.3.1 Morphological sequences

In the past, uninjected T2- and T1-weighted sequences in breast MRI were not considered very useful, due to their low diagnostic value. Since then, many authors have demonstrated the value of using morphological sequences.

T2-weighted sequences can be used to detect cystic lesions whose presence indicates benign enhancement, whether annular enhancement in inflammatory cysts or non-mass enhancement in fibrocystic mastopathy.

T2-weighted sequences with fat saturation are very useful in the case of nipple discharge, enabling indirect MRI galactography images to be created, and also improve the detection of small cancers (fig. 21).

T1-weighted sequences without fat saturation are useful for detecting the presence of a fatty component in a lesion, an important factor in favor of benignity (fig. 22). These sequences are also useful for confirming the correct position of metal markers in the biopsy site [46] (fig. 23).

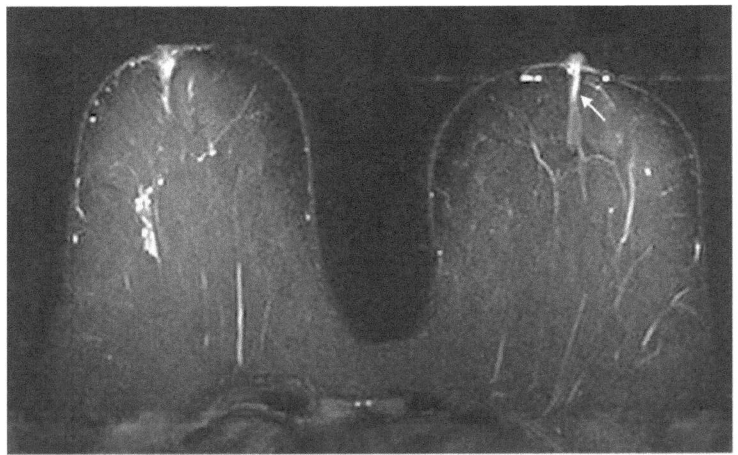

Fig. 21. Ductal ectasia. Intracanal hypersignal on T2 sequences with fat supression (arrows).

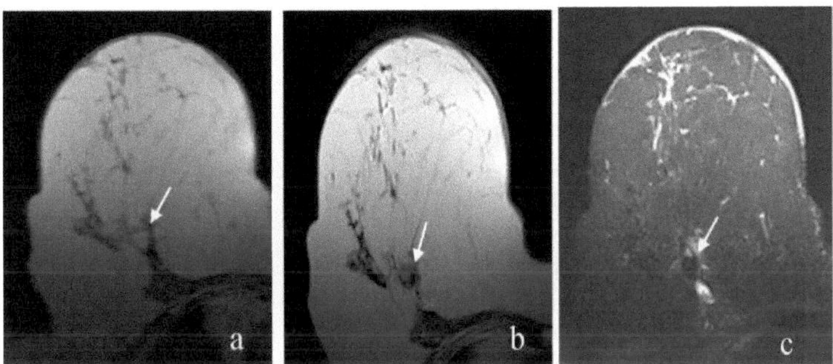

Fig. 22 Cytosteatonecrosis: (a) T1 sequence, (b) T2 sequence, (c) T2 Fat Sat sequence. Lesion in T1 hypersignal, T2 hypersignal, hyposignal on T2 sequence with fat supression (arrows).

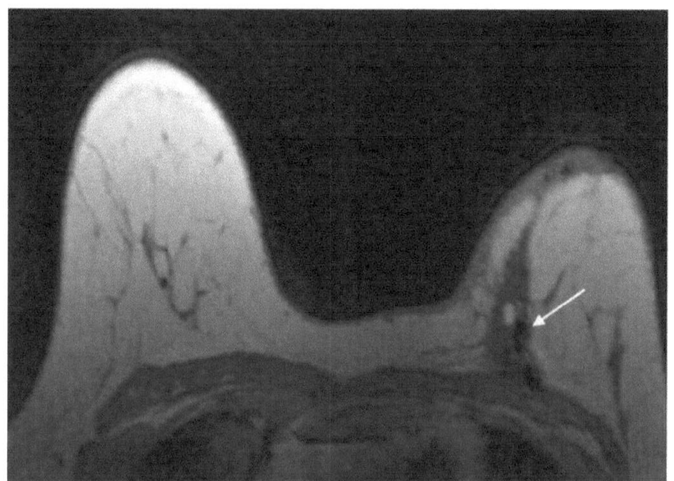

Fig. 23. Position of metal marker in ground on T1 sequence (arrow).

3.5.3.2 Dynamic sequences

Dynamic analysis makes it possible to distinguish suspicious abnormal angiogenesis among the various enhancement kinetics. T1 gradient echo sequences after injection of gadolinium chelate (fig. 24).

2D or 3D acquisition?

Compared with 2D sequences, 3D sequences give finer slices with a better signal-to-noise ratio [43]. On the other hand, as 3D acquisition is performed without fat suppression, it is desirable to use 2D sequences to reduce phase-encoding artifacts that extend in all three directions in 3D sequences, masking contours and making it difficult to detect these artifacts on subtraction sequences.

The 3D sequence enables volume analysis of the lesion (measurement in 3 planes, distance from the nipple-areolar plate and the deep pectoral plane).

3.5.3.3 Complementary sequences

• **Broadcast**

The principle of diffusion imaging is to quantify the movement of water molecules in tissues. The objectives of diffusion sequences are to optimize detection of small lesions and improve characterization of benign and malignant lesions. Diffusion MRI can also be used to assess response to neoadjuvant chemotherapy. An increase of more than 10% in ADC coefficients at the end of the first cycle of chemotherapy signifies a decrease in cell density, and is therefore predictive of response to treatment [47, 48].

• **Magnetic resonance spectroscopy**

Spectroscopy is a molecular imaging technique. Its principle is to highlight an abnormal choline peak in malignant tumors (resonance at 3.2 ppm) [49]. Bartella et al. reported that the addition of spectroscopy to the standard protocol improved the PPV of biopsies from 35% to 82% (p < 0.01), and enabled biopsy to be avoided in 57% of lesions [50]. In addition, numerous studies have shown that this sequence can demonstrate an early response (at 24 h) to neoadjuvant chemotherapy [51].

The three types of spectroscopic enhancement curves described by CK. Kuhl et al [52]:

- Type I: an initial slow, then progressive enhancement curve (fig. 25)

- Type II: a rapid initial enhancement curve, followed by a plateau (fig. 26).

- Type III: a rapid initial enhancement curve, followed by a washout (fig. 27).

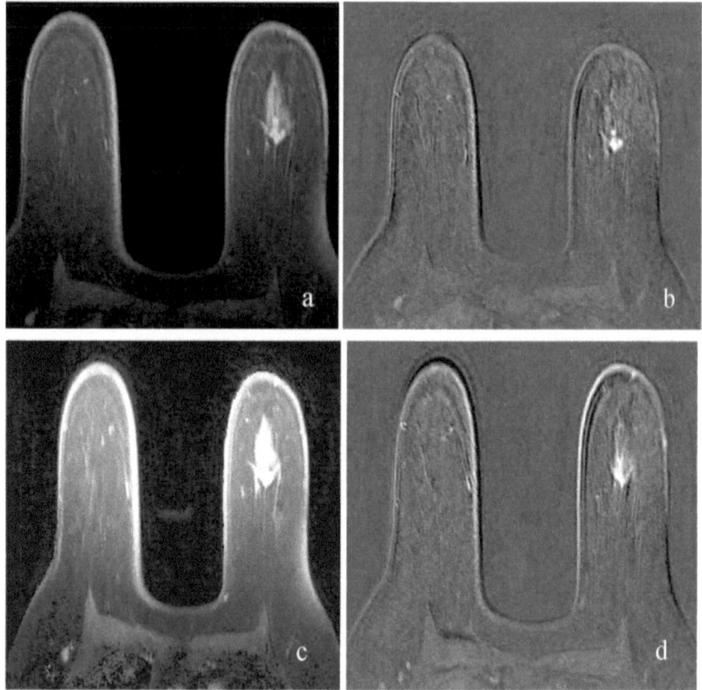

Fig. 24. Enhancement analysis of a malignant tumor of the left breast.

Dynamic analysis enables the tumor to be distinguished from the rest of the fibroglandular parenchyma thanks to acquisition before the second minute in three-dimensional (3D) T1 weighting (a) and 3D T1 injected with subtraction (b). At six minutes, it is difficult to differentiate the cancer from the breast parenchyma on T1 3D injected (c) and T1 3D injected with subtraction (d) sequences.

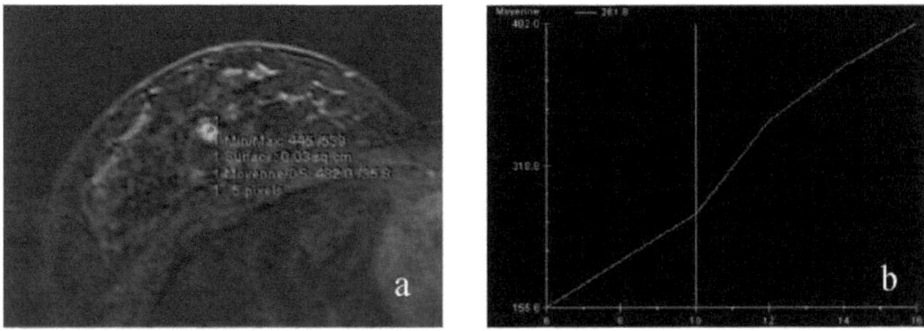

Fig. 25. Type I curve. (a) Subtracted injected sequences, axial section. (b) Enhancement curve. Histology: fibroadenoma.

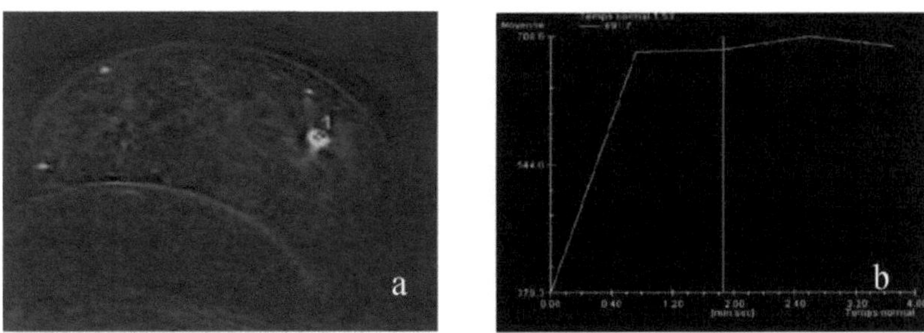

Fig. 26 Type II curve: (a) Subtracted injected sequences, axial section. (b) Enhancement curve. Histology: fibroadenoma.

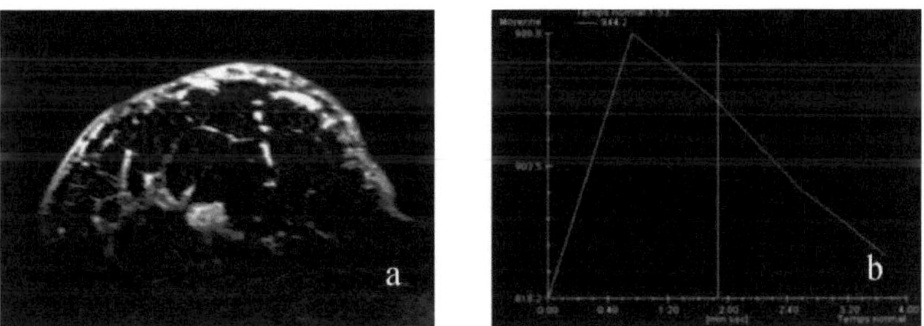

Fig. 27. Type III curve: (a) Subtracted injected sequences, axial section. (b) Enhancement curve. Histology: Invasive lobular carcinoma.

Anatomy - imaging correlations

1. Mammography [9, 53, 54]

Mammography produces a two-dimensional projection of the breast. The mammographic image is a superimposition of all the tissues making up the breast, varying according to the proportion of the different constituents (parenchymal tissue, adipose tissue, connective tissue), age and hormonal impregnation.

The different elements visualized by mammography, from surface to depth.

1.1. The skin covering

The cutaneous plane is a dense border, approximately 1 mm thick (fig. 28); it is thicker at the areola and in the sub-mammary region. Skin pores may be visible as punctiform blisters.

1.2. The nipple

The nipple is dense on mammography, cylindrical-conical in shape, about 1cm long and should be located outside the contours of the gland (fig. 28). The nipple may become invaginated or hypertrophied.

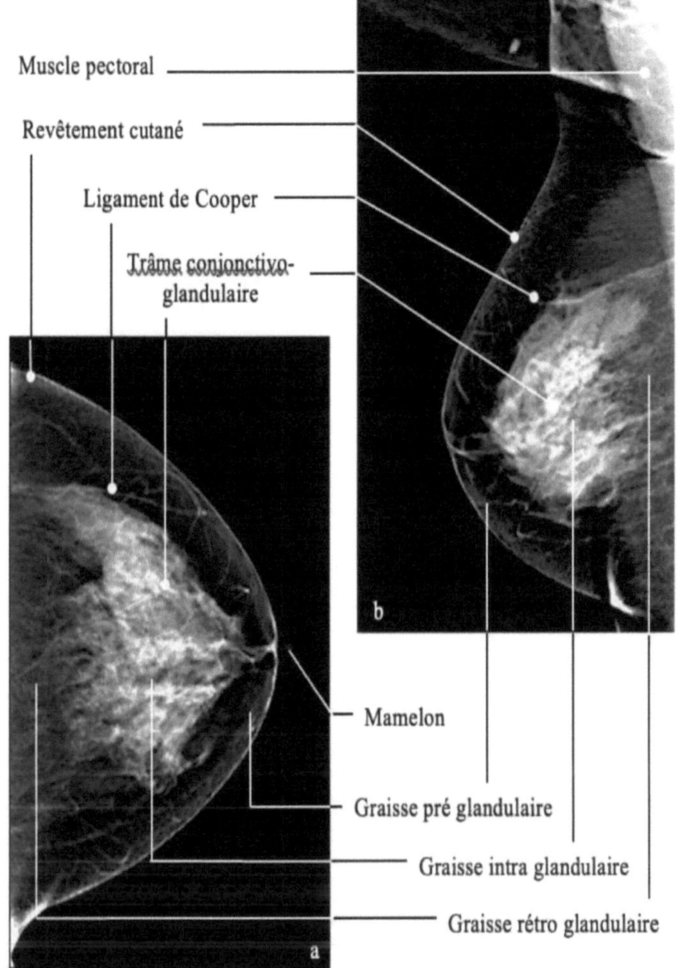

Fig. 28. Breast constitution. Mammography, (a) craniocaudal incidence, (b) oblique incidence.

1.3. Glandular tissue

Imaging of the breast contents depends on the glandular component. Lobular elements are visible thanks to the contrast of the intralobular connective tissue and, on mammography, appear as small, fuzzy micronodular opacities [55]. Galactophore ducts are not spontaneously visible on mammography, except in the case of very fatty environments and ductal dilatation (fig. 29).

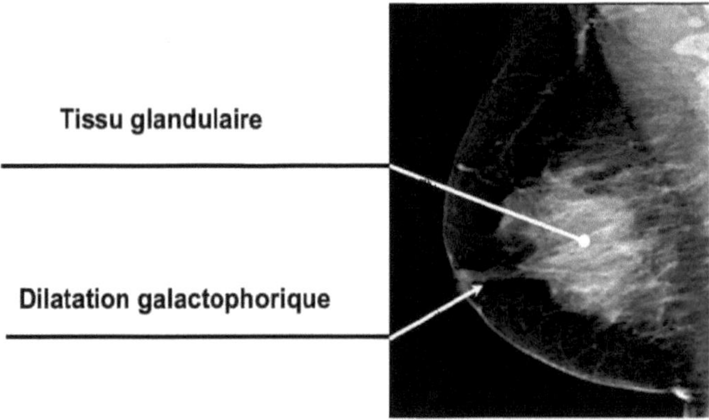

Fig. 29. Galactophoric dilatation. Mammography, incidence

1.4. Connective tissue

The connective tissue, radiopaque, is sparse and its opacity is confused with that of the glandular tissue. Cooper's ligaments appear as linear or arciform opacities. They are generally visible on oblique or profile mammography. Cooper's ligaments are prominent in subcutaneous adipose tissue, along the upper edge of the parenchyma (fig. 28).

1.5. Adipose tissue

Adipose tissue, radiolucent on mammography. A subcutaneous,

preglandular fatty space is crossed by Cooper's ligaments, and a retroglandular fatty space separates the gland from the pectoral muscle and should not contain any glandular tissue. This is the *no-man's-land* zone described by Tabar [55,56] (fig. 28).

1.6. The muscles

On the craniocaudal view, the pectoral muscle is inconsistently projected forward of the chest wall in the form of a half-moon. On the medio-lateral oblique view, the pectoralis muscle is seen as a concave structure behind the retroglandular fat (fig. 28).

The sternal muscle is located in internal projection on craniocaudal incidence, rarely visible in 1% of patients (fig. 30).

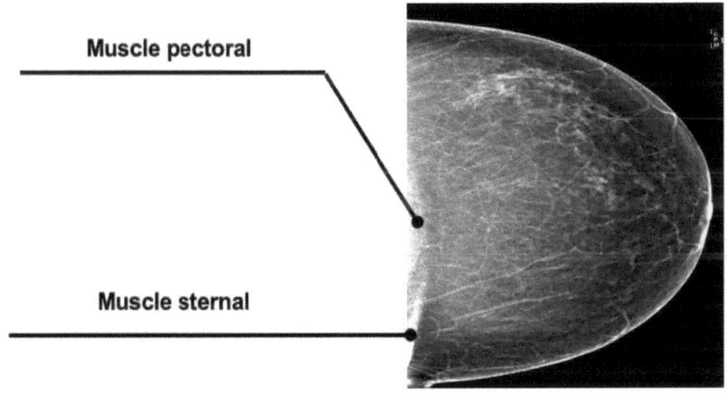

Fig. 30. Visualization of the sternal muscle projection. Mammography, frontal view.

1.7. Vessels

Vessels can be visualized, especially if the contrast is fatty. They appear as dense, ribbon-like structures. Veins are larger than arteries. Occasionally, vessels can be identified by atheromatous parietal calcifications (fig. 31).

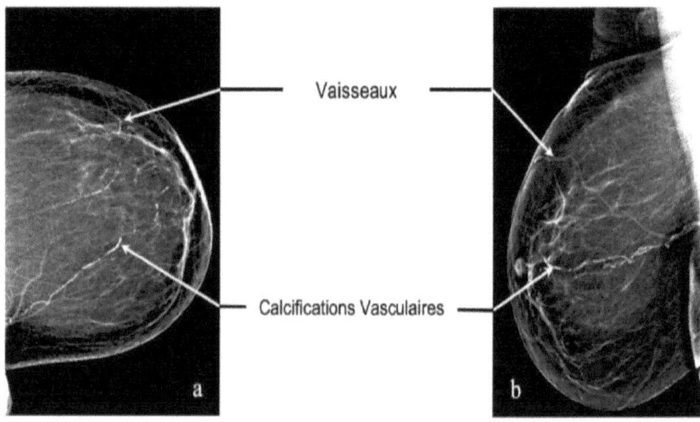

Fig. 31. Vascularization. (a) Mammography, craniocaudal incidence, (b) oblique incidence.

1.8. Lymphatic vessels

Lymphatic vessels are absent in normal breasts. Lymph nodes are detected intra-mammary in 5% of normal mammograms [57] (fig. 32). They have the appearance of a kidney-shaped or dense coffee-bean structure with a clear fat center, and are usually located along the vessels (fig. 32).

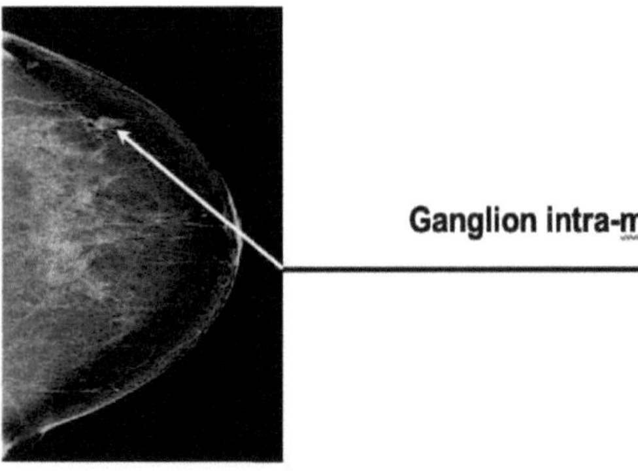

Fig. 32. Intramammary ganglion, with clear center, projecting from a vascular structure. Mammogram, frontal view.

The different mammographic aspects result from the variable proportion between fibrous and fatty elements in the breast. The earliest classification was described by Wolfe in 1967 [58], determining four types of glandular density (N1, P1, P2, NY), with type N1 corresponding to a totally fatty glandular structure through to type NY, which corresponds to a totally dense glandular structure. The American College of Radiology has adapted these different categories in Breast Imaging Reporting into 4 types from "a" to "d" [59], (appendix 1) (fig. 33).

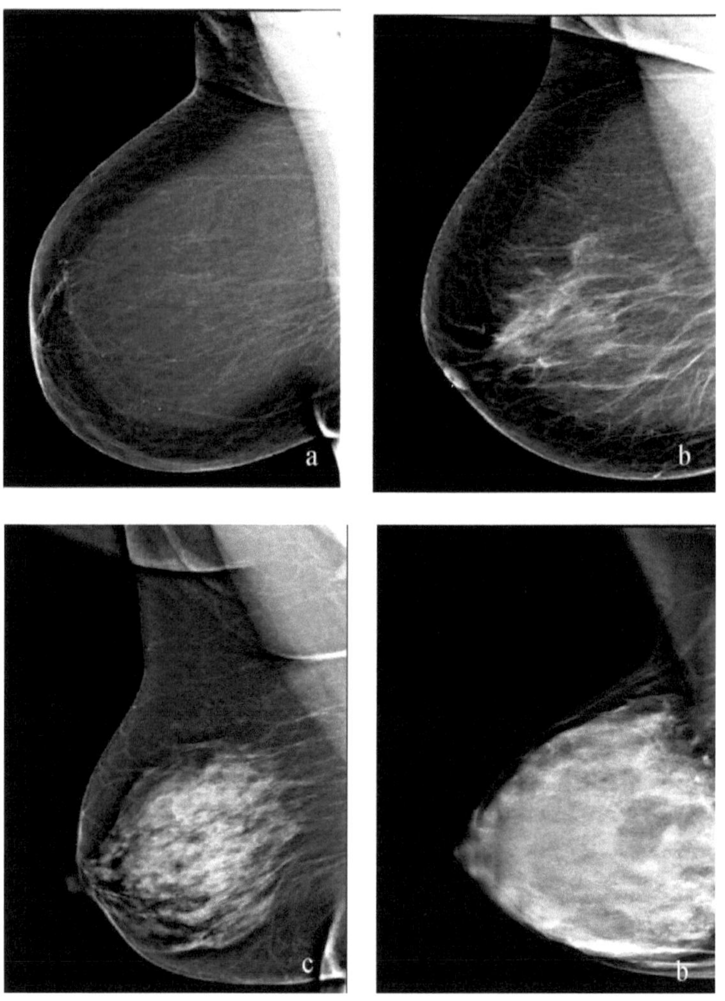

Fig. 33. Breast density according to ACR BI-RADS classification.
Mammography, oblique incidence. (a): almost entirely fatty, type a; (b): scattered patches of fibroglandular tissue, type b; (c): heterogeneous dense breast, type c; (d): extremely dense breast, type d.

2. Ultrasonography [6,7, 9, 54, 60-62]

Several sonographic aspects are encountered, depending on the proportion of adipose tissue, fibroglandular tissue and ductal elements. This aspect may also vary according to the glandular sector being analyzed. In adult women, we find the following elements from surface to depth:

2.1. The skin covering

Skin thickness varies from 0.5 to 2 mm. It is visualized on ultrasound as a double echogenic line separated by a thin hypoechoic border (fig.

34)   . These lines merge at the nipple-areolar plate.

2.2. The nipple

The nipple is a hypoechoic structure which may be responsible for ultrasound attenuation, in which case the probe must be obliquely positioned to explore the retroareolar region (fig. 34).

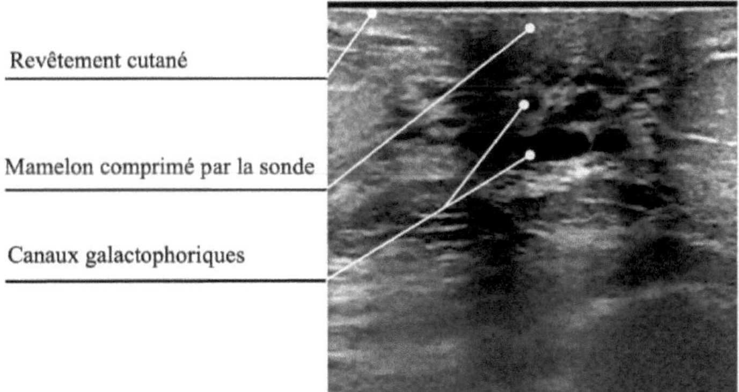

Fig. 34. ultrasound section centred on the nipple.

2.3. Glandular tissue

The echogenicity of glandular parenchyma varies with age and individual composition. In young women and during pregnancy and lactation, glandular tissue is often hypoechoic and homogeneous; during genital activity, glandular parenchyma is hyperechoic and homogeneous, with variable thickness. With age, breast parenchyma becomes heterogeneous due to fatty involution, the echostructure is hypoechoic interspersed with hyperechoic areas corresponding to connective fibers and residual parenchyma. When fibrous involution predominates, the echostructure is hyperechoic and heterogeneous.

The ACR BI-RADS classification describes three basic types of echostructure (fig. 35) :

- type a: homogeneous fatty echostructure with fat lobules and echogenic bands of Cooper's ligaments, with no echogenic zones in the area analysed ;
- type b: homogeneous, uniformly echogenic fibroglandular ;
- type c: heterogeneous fibroglandular, heterogeneity may be focal or diffuse (Appendix 2).

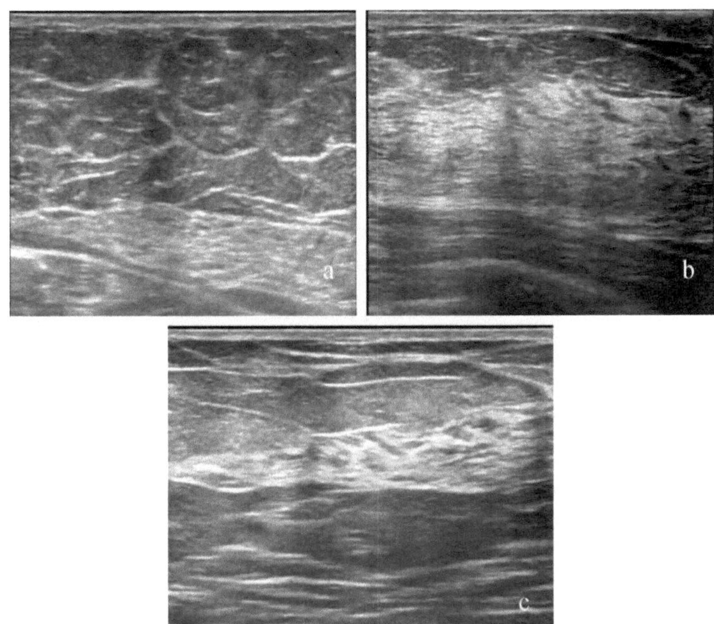

Fig. 35. Echostructure according to ACR BI-RADS lexicon.

Ultrasound.

(a)   homogeneous fat echostructure ;

(b)   homogeneous fibroglandular echostructure ;

(c)   heterogeneous echostucture (focal or diffuse).

2.4. Connective tissue

Connective tissue is hyperechoic, often confused with glandular tissue. Cooper's ligaments are hyperechoic, crossing the layer of subcutaneous fatty tissue and appearing as thin, uniformly echogenic bands (fig. 36).

2.5. Adipose tissue

Subcutaneous fat appears as a hypoechoic line of variable thickness, partitioned by triangular hyperechoic structures representing Duret's ridges, the attachment zone of Cooper's ligaments. Intraglandular fatty tissue appears as well-limited oblong hypoechoic areas. In the supine position, the thickness of the retromammary fatty space is reduced, in contrast to the mammographic appearance. This fatty space appears as a homogeneous hypoechoic band (fig. 36).

2.6. The muscles

The muscle planes appear as echogenic lamellar structures (fig. 36)   .

2.7. Ribs

The ribs are seen as hyperechoic, attenuating arciform structures (fig. 36).

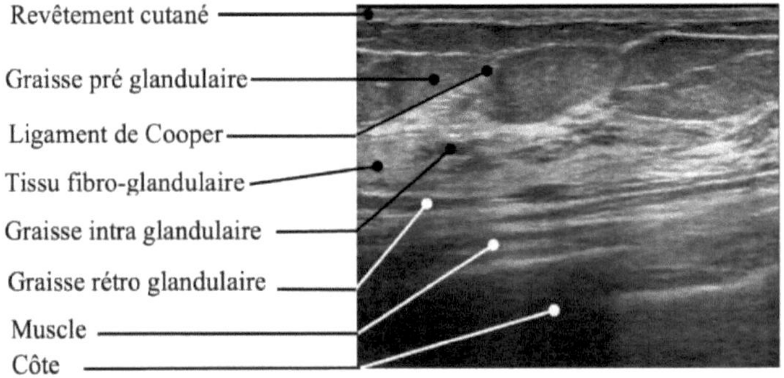

Fig. 36. Breast constitution. Ultrasound.

2.8. Vessels

Axillary vessels appear as hypoechoic tubular structures. They are best analyzed in Doppler mode. Intra-breast vessels are sometimes visible in Doppler mode (fig. 37).

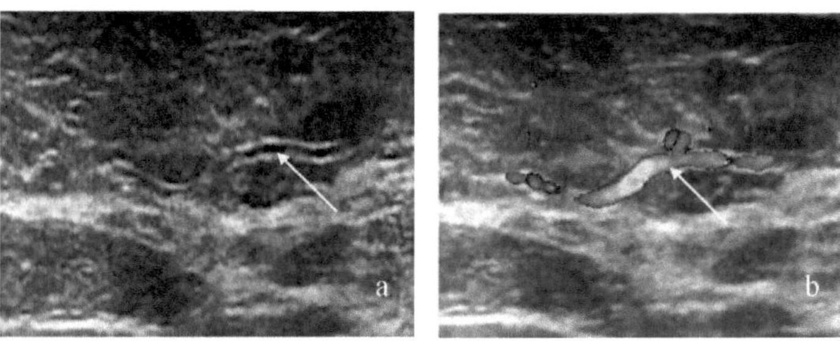

Fig. 37. Intramammary vessels. (a) Ultrasound. Tubular structure

2.9. Lymphatic vessels

Lymphatic vessels are absent in a normal breast. Nodes appear as kidney-shaped or coffee-bean structures with hypoechoic cortex and hyperechoic fatty hilum (fig. 38).

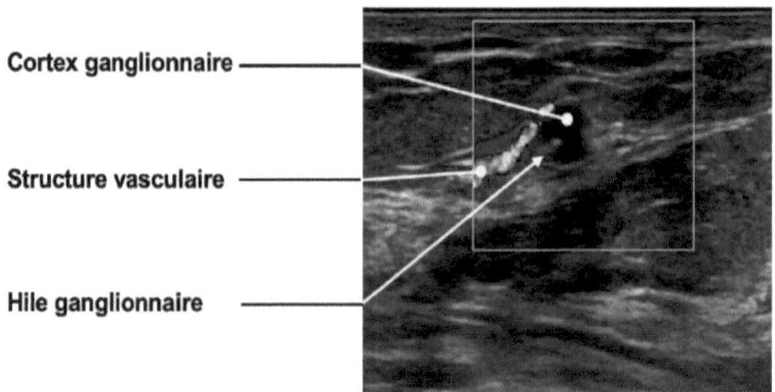

Fig. 38. Intramammary ganglion. Doppler ultrasound. Hypoechoic ganglion cortex and hyperechoic fatty ganglion hilum, presenting on a vascular pathway.

3. MRI

Breast anatomy can be demonstrated very well with breast MRI. It can be used to evaluate deep areas of the breast, such as the deep muscles and chest wall. Certain structures, such as vessels and lymph nodes, are easily visible, especially after contrast injection. Knowledge of the normal anatomy of the breast on MRI is fundamental to the correct interpretation of the examination.

3.1. The nipple

Contrast enhancement of the nipple is present in 50% of cases [9] and should not be considered pathological in the absence of suggestive clinical signs. These enhancements sometimes extend to the retro-nipple region, and the bilateral nature of these images confirms their normality (fig. 39).

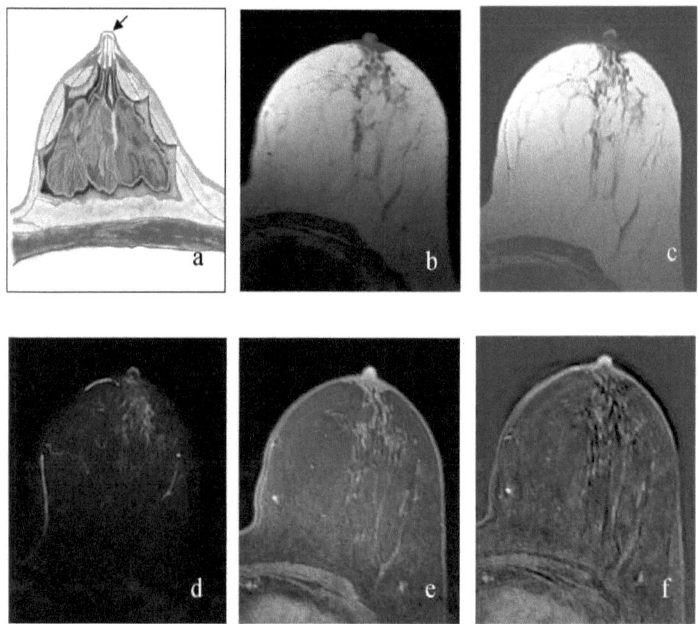

Fig. 39. Nipple. (a) Diagram (arrow). (b) T1-weighted sequence. (c) T2-weighted sequence. (d) T2 Fat Sat sequence. (e) T1 Fat Sat injected sequence. (f) Subtracted injected sequence.

3.2. Galactophore ducts

Galactophore ducts are not spontaneously visible, except in the case of galactophore ectasia, which are visualized as retroareolar ductal structures converging towards the nipple, with a variable signal depending on their content (fig. 40).

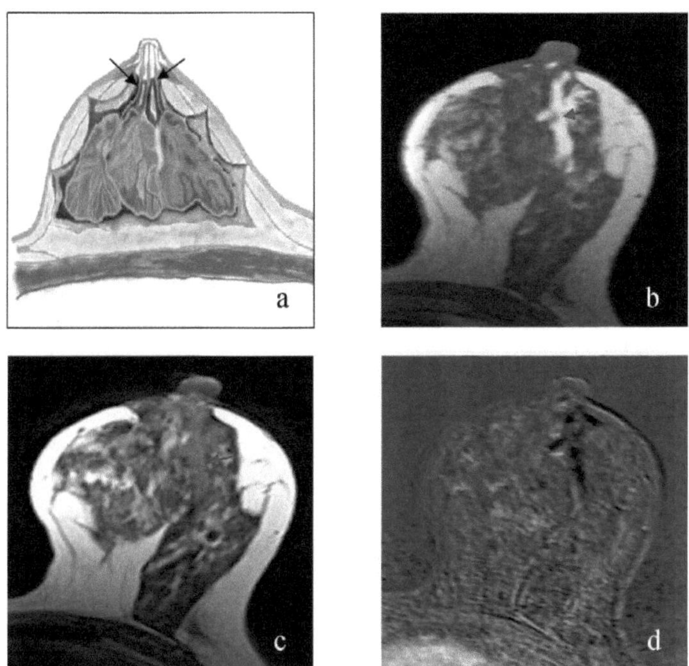

Fig. 40. Galactophoric dilatation (a) Diagram (arrows). (b) T1-weighted sequence. (c) T2-weighted sequence. (d) Injected subtraction sequence. Protein-containing ductal ectasia in T1 hypersignal, T2 hyposignal, unenhanced after contrast injection (arrows).

3.3. Adipose tissue

Adipose tissue appears hypersignal on T1- and T2-weighted sequences, TSE T2 hyposignal with fat suppression and unenhanced after intravenous injection of contrast medium (fig. 41). Subcutaneous fat is partitioned by the suspensory ligaments of the breast, known as Cooper's ligaments, in the extension of Duret's fibro-glandular ridges.

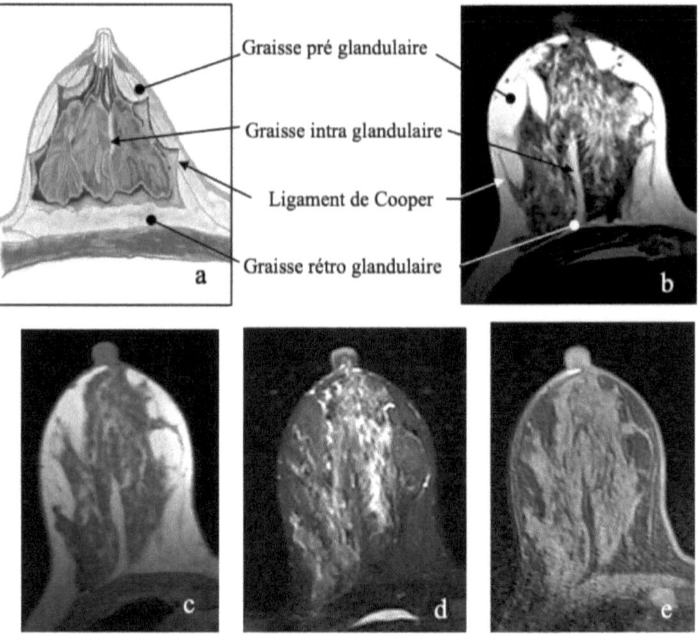

Fig. 41. Adipose tissue (a) Diagram. (b) T2-weighted sequence. (c) T1-weighted sequence. (d) T2 Fat Sat sequence. (e) T1 Fat Sat injected sequence. adipose tissue in T2 and T1 hypersignal, unenhanced after contrast injection.

3.4. Fibro-glandular tissue

Fibro-glandular tissue is a normal component of the breast. It can be assessed on T1- and T2-weighted sequences, and should be quantified according to the BIRADS lexicon into four categories [59]: A. Fatty breast; B. Scattered fibro-glandular tissue; C. Heterogeneous fibro-glandular tissue; D. Dense fibro-glandular tissue (fig. 42).

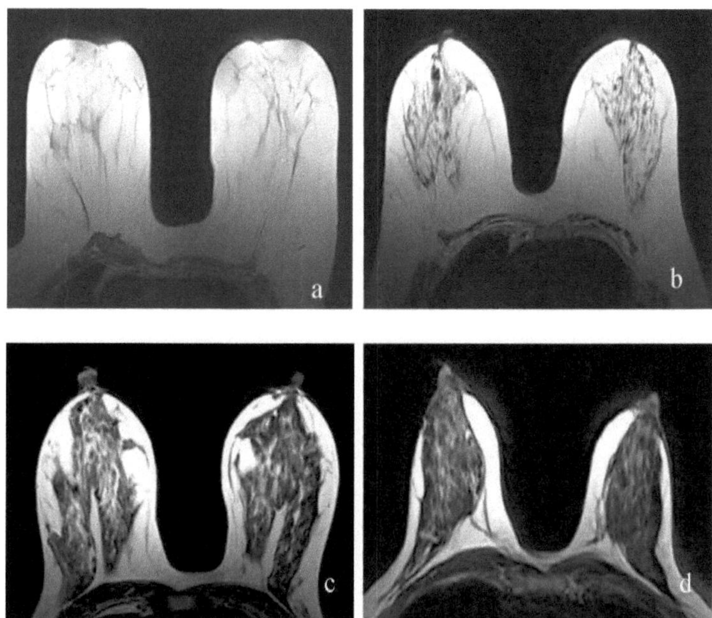

Fig. 42. Breast density according to ACR BI-RADS classification. T2-weighted sequences. (a): Fatty breast, type A; (b): Scattered fibro-glandular tissue, type B; (c): Heterogeneous fibro-glandular tissue, type C; (d): Dense fibro-glandular tissue, type D.

On fat-suppressed T1 sequences and after injection of gadolinium chelate, fibro-glandular tissue may be enhanced. This physiological enhancement can be described according to the BIRADS lexicon in four levels: A. minimal; B. slight; C. moderate, and D. marked (fig. 43).

Matrix enhancement is assessed 90 seconds after injection, at the moment when malignant lesions are enhanced, to determine whether this matrix enhancement may be masking cancer. In general, matrix enhancement is progressive and may extend throughout the breast. However, it is plausible to observe very early, rapid and intense fibro-glandular enhancement.

Whatever the phase of the cycle, matrix enhancement is possible and may persist after the menopause.

Matrix enhancement is not directly related to the amount of glandular tissue. A patient with dense breasts may show little or no matrix enhancement. On the other hand, a patient with sparse fibro-glandular tissue may have marked matrix enhancement. The level of matrix enhancement should be reported in the case report.

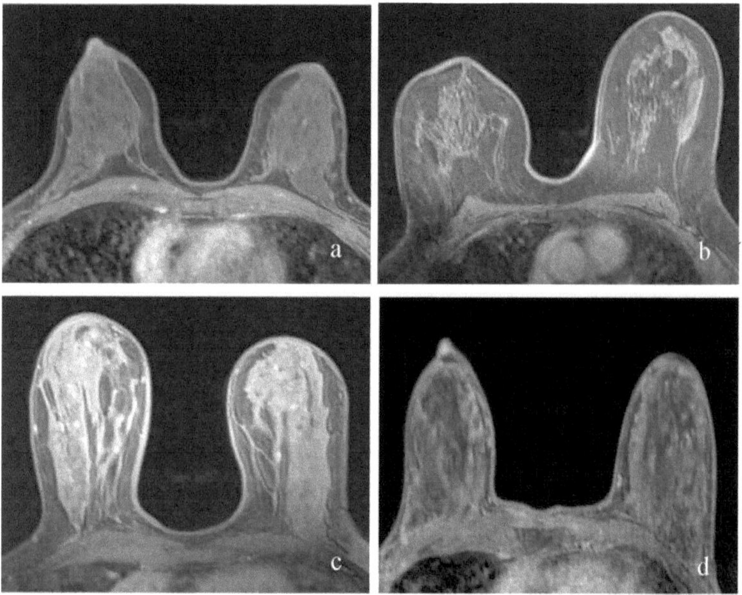

Fig. 43. Physiological enhancement of fibroglandular breast tissue. T1 sequences injected with fat suppression in four levels according to the BIRADS lexicon: minimal (a), slight (b), moderate (c) and marked (d).

3.5. Muscles

Muscles appear intermediate on morphological T1 and T2 sequences.

Muscles are weakly enhanced after contrast injection. Axial and sagittal sections clearly show the posterior adipose-muscle interface, revealing its integrity or its involvement by posterior cancers (fig. 44).

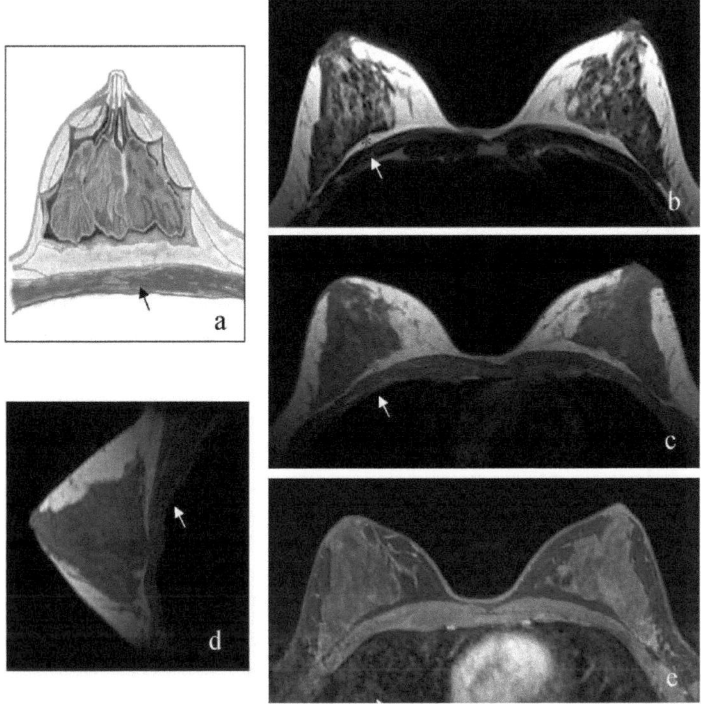

Fig. 44. Pectoral muscle. (a) Diagram (b) T2-weighted sequence. (c+d) T1-weighted sequence, axial section (c), sagittal section (d). (e) Native T1-injected sequence. The pectoralis muscle is in intermediate T2 and T1 signal, weakly enhanced after contrast injection (arrow). Posterior adipomuscular interface (asterisk).

3.6. Vessels

The lateral thoracic artery arises from the axillary artery and supplies the upper outer quadrant of the breast, accounting for around 30% of the breast vascularization (fig. 4). Sixty percent of the mammary vascularization comes from the internal mammary artery and its perforating branches, which supply the central and internal part of the breast (fig. 4). The remainder of the vascular supply comes mainly from branches of the intercostal arteries. Vessels are easily identified, and may be visible along part of their course in the slice, or follow their course in several successive slices. Maximum intensity projection (MIP) images can also help confirm vessel trajectories (fig. 45).

The spontaneous signal of vessels, particularly in T2, and their enhancement are variable. These variations are linked to the flow velocity within the vessel and its orientation in relation to the slice plane.

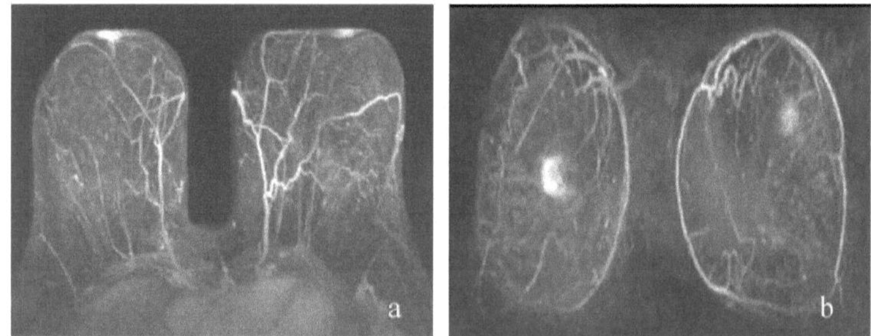

Fig. 45. Maximum intensity projection (MIP) reconstruction. (a) Axial section. (b) Coronal section.

3.7. Lymph nodes

Lymphatic drainage of the breast is mainly from lateral and medial trunks extending from the areola to the axilla (97%), with the internal mammary chain accounting for the remaining 3% [63]. Berg's level I lymph nodes are located below the pectoralis minor muscle. Level II lymph nodes are located behind the pectoralis minor muscle, and level III lymph nodes are located above the pectoralis minor muscle (fig. 5).

Nodes are encountered in most MRI scans. Their topography is usually behind or in the external extension of the pectoralis major muscle. Intramammary nodes are easily diagnosed with their reniform appearance, with sharp, regular contours, in T1 and T2 hyposignal, and their fatty hilum in T1 and T2 hypersignal. Contrast enhancement is usually early, rapid and moderate (fig. 46). However, lymph nodes can present a diagnostic dilemma [64] when morphological criteria are not typical. The dynamic curve may be unreliable, often mimicking malignant lesions. T2-weighted images with fat suppression may be useful in these cases, as the signal intensity of the nodes is greater than that of normal glandular parenchyma.

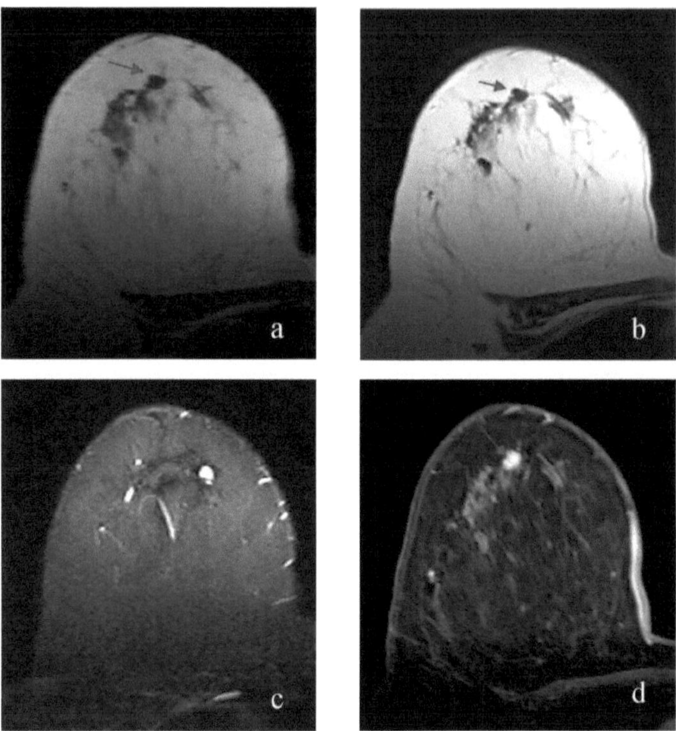

Fig. 46. Intramammary ganglion. (a) T1-weighted sequence (b) T2-weighted sequence (c) T2 Fat Sat sequence (d) T1 injected sequence. Reniform intramammary ganglion, with sharp, regular contours, in T1 and T2 hyposignal, T2 Fat Sat hyper signal and enhanced after contrast injection with a fatty hilum in T1 and T2 hypersignal (arrows).

Appendices

Appendix 1: Bi-Rads® mammography evaluation categories

BI-RADS 0: Incomplete assessment requiring further imaging

BI-RADS 1: Normal mammography

BI-RADS 2: Benign abnormality.

BI-RADS 3: Anomaly probably benign, with a risk of malignancy < 2%, short-term monitoring is recommended.

BI-RADS 4: Suspicious abnormality, with a probability of malignancy of between 3% and 95%, requiring histological analysis.
4a = low probability,
4b = moderate probability,
4c = high probability.

BI-RADS 5: Highly suspicious anomaly, with probability of malignancy > 95%, requiring surgical removal.

BI-RADS 6: Known histological result: proven malignancy.

Appendix 2: Bi-Rads® ultrasound evaluation categories

BI-RADS 0: Incomplete assessment, requiring further tests.

BI-RADS 1: Examination considered strictly normal

BI-RADS 2: Benign lesion(s): Simple cysts, intra-mammary lymph nodes, breast implants, stable post-surgical changes, stable probable fibroadenomas.

BI-RADS 3: Anomaly probably benign. Short-term surveillance suggested. For example: solid masses with circumscribed contours, oval, parallel orientation (probable fibroadenoma), complicated cysts that cannot be palpated, clusters of microcysts.

BI-RADS 4: Suspicious abnormality, with a probability of malignancy between 2 and 95%, requiring histological analysis.

- 4a = low probability $\geq$ 2% to < 10%,

- 4b = moderate probability $\geq$ 10% to < 50%,

- 4c = high probability $\geq$ 50 to < 95%.

BI-RADS 5: Highly suspicious anomaly with > 95% probability of malignancy, requiring surgical removal.

BI-RADS 6: Known histological findings, proven malignancy

References

1. Boisserie-Lacroix M, Bokobsa J, Boutet G, Colle M, Hocké C, Le Treut A. Sénologie de l'enfant et de l'adolescente Médecine-Sciences Flammarion éd, Paris, 1998, 183 p.

2. Couturaud B, Fitoussi A. Anatomy/surgery of breast cancer. Conservative treatment, oncoplasty. Techniques chirurgicales gynécologie. Elsevier Masson; 2011; 4-7.

3. Chopier J, Jalaguier-Coudray A, Thomassin-Naggara I. Variations of the normal breast. Mammographic and ultrasonographic aspects. EMC - RADIOLOGIE ET IMAGERIE MEDICALE : Génito-urinaire - Gynéco-obstétricale - Mammaire 2011:1-16 [Article 34-800-A-15].

4. Brigitte M, Kamina P; Anatomie chirurgical du sein Cancer du sein. Elsevier Masson; 2007; 2-10.

5. Cardiff, R. D. and S. R. Wellings. "The comparative pathology of humanand mouse mammary glands." J Mammary Gland Biol Neoplasia; 1999; 4: 105-22.

6. Levy L. The normal breast and its variants: breast cancers. Mammography and Mammary Ultrasound 2006.

7. Cartier JM, Bourjat P. The normal breast. Imagerie du sein : La pratique sénologique quotidienne 1998 ; 33-35.

8. Kopans DB. Anatomy, histology, physiology and pathology: In Breast imaging. Philadelphia. Lippincott-Raven Publishers 1998; 3-27.

9. Heywang-Kobrunner S H, Schreer I, Bassler R, Perlet C, Viehweg P. Normal breast. Imagerie diagnostique du sein : Mammographie, échographie, IRM, techniques interventionnelles 2007 ; 183-202.

10. Garbay JR. Anatomy of the breast and axillary region. Breast Cancer

Surgery: Diagnostic, Curative and Reconstructive 1997; 3-17.

11. Berg JW.The significance of axillary node levels in the study of breast carcinoma.Cancer, 1955; 8: 776-8.

12. McNally, S. & Martin, F. Molecular regulators of pubertal mammary gland development. Ann. Med. 43, 212 R 34; 2011.

13. Kamina P. Anatomie gynecologique et obstetricale. Paris ; Maloine ; 1984 ; P459 ; 469 ; 471-476; 513.

14. Austin C. R and Short R. V. Hormonal Control of Reproduction. 2nd edition of Reproduction in Mammals, Vol.3. Cambridge : Cambridge University Press. 1984.

15. Baur A, Bahrs SD, Speck S, Wietek BM, Kremer B, Vogel U, et al. Breast MRI of pure ductal carcinoma in situ: sensitivity of diagnosis and influence of lesion characteristics. Eur J Radiol 2013;82:1731-7.

16. Hammcrslcya JA, Partridgeb SC, Blitzera GC, Deitcha S, Rahbarb II. Management of high-risk breast lesions found on mammogram or ultrasound: the value of contrast-enhanced MRI to exclude malignancy. Clinical Imaging 49; 2018; 174180.

17. Andolina VF, Lillé SL, Willison KM, Mammographic Imaging. A pratical guide. 2 nd ed. Lippincott Williams and Wilkins; 2001.

18. Austin C. R and Short R. V. Hormonal Control of Reproduction. 2nd edition of Reproduction in Mammals, Vol.3. Cambridge : Cambridge University Press. 1984.

19. Faulconer LS, Parham CA, Connor DM, Kuzmiak C, et al. Effect of breast compression on lesion characteristic visibility with diffraction-enhanced imaging. Acad Radiol 2010; 17 (4) : 433-40. Epub 2009 Dec 29.

20. Kinzelin S. Positioning, the key step in mammography examination. Imagerie du sein Elsevier Masson, 2012; 2: 19-27.

21. Mancuso S, Ottolenghi G. The oblique projection in the radiologic Study of the breast. Minerva Ginecol 1989; 41 (7): 325-8.

22. Konguth PJ, Rimer BK, Conaway MR, et al. Impact of patient-controlled compression on the mammography experience. Radiology 1993; 186 (1) : 99-102.

23. Muntz EP, Logan WW, Focal spot size. And scatter supression in magnification mammography. AJR Am J Roentgenol 1979; 133 (3) : 453-9.

24. Corsetti V, Houssami N, Ferrari A, Ghirardi M, Bellarosa S, Angelini O, et al. Breast screening with ultrasound in women with mammography-negative dense breasts: evidence on incremental cancer detection and false positives, and associated cost. Eur J Cancer. 2008 Mar;44(4):539-44.

25. Athanasiou A, Tardivon A, Ollivier L, Thibault F, El Khoury C, Neuenschwander S. How to optimize breast ultrasound. Eur J Radiol. 2009 Jan;69(1):6-13.

26. Weinstein SP, Conant EF, Sehgal C. Technical advances in breast ultrasound imaging. Semin Ultrasound CT MR. 2006 Aug;27(4):273-83.

2 7. Sehgal CM, Weinstein SP, Arger PH, Conant EF. A review of breast ultrasound. J Mammary Gland Biol Neoplasia. 2006 Apr;11(2):113-23.

28. Amersham Health. Encyclopaedia of Medical Imaging. http://eu.aershamhealth/com/medcyclopaedia/

29. Clevert DA, Jung EM, Jungius KP, Ertan K, Kubale R. Value of tissue harmonic imaging (THI) and contrast harmonic imaging (CHI) in

detection and characterisation of breast tumours. Eur Radiol 2007 ; 17 : 1-10.

30. Rosen EL, Soo MS. Tissue harmonic imaging sonography of breast lesions: improved margin analysis, conspicuity, and image quality compared to conventional ultrasound. Clin Imaging. 2001 Nov-Dec;25(6):379-84.

31. Athanasiou A, Balleyguier C. New techniques in breast ultrasound. Imagerie de la Femme. 2007;17(4):247-54.

32. Huber S, Wagner M, Medl M, Czembirek H. Real-time spatial compound imaging in breast ultrasound. Ultrasound Med Biol 2002 ; 28 : 155-63.

33. Cha JH, Moon WK, Cho N, Chung SY, Park SH, Park JM, et al. Differentiation of benign from malignant solid breast masses: conventional US versus compound imaging. Radiology 2005;237:841-6.

34. Balu-Maestro C. Basics of breast ultrasound. Imager ie du sein. Paris : Elsevier-Masson ; 2012. p. 101-17.

35. Dickinson RJ, Hill CR. Measurement of soft tissue motion using correlation between A-scans.Ultrasound Med Biol 1982;8(3):263-71.

36. Krouskop TA, Dougherty DR, Vinson FS. A pulsed Doppler ultrasonic system for making noninvasive measurements of the mechanical properties of soft tissue. J Rehabil Res Dev 1987;24(2):1-8.

37. Youk JH, Gweon HM, Son EJ. Shear-wave elastography in breast ultrasonography: the state of the art. Ultrasonography. 2017 Oct;36(4):300-309. doi: 10.14366/usg.17024.

38. Tristant H, Benmussa M, Bokobsa J, Elbaz P. Variation of the normal breast: mammographic and ultrasonographic aspects. Encycl Méd Chir 1994; 810-G-15.

3 9. Sardanelli F, Boetes C, Borisch B, Decker T, Federico M, Gilbert FJ, et al. Magnetic resonance imaging of the breast: recommendations from the EUSOMA working group. Eur J Cancer. 2010 May;46(8):1296-316.

40. El Khouli RH, Macura KJ, Kamel IR, Bluemke DA, Jacobs MA. The effects of applying breast compression in dynamic contrast material-enhanced MR imaging. Radiology 2014;272:79-90.

41. Wilkinson J, Appleton CM, Margenthaler JA. Utility of breast MRI for evaluation of residual disease following excisional biopsy. J Surg Res 2011;170:233-9.

42. Lee JM, Orel SG, Czerniecki BJ, Solin LJ, Schnall MD. MRI before reexcision surgery in patients with breast cancer. AJR Am J Roentgenol 2004;182:473-80.

4 3. Orel SG, Reynolds C, Schnall MD, Solin LJ, Fraker DL, Sullivan DC. Breast carcinoma:MRimaging before re-excisional biopsy. Radiology 1997;205:429-36.

44. Kuhl C. The current status of breast MR imaging. Part I. Choice of technique, image interpretation, diagnostic accuracy, and transfer to clinical practice. Radiology. 2007 Aug;244(2):356-78.

45. Mann RM,Kuhl CK, Kinkel K, Boetes C. Breast MRI: guidelines from the European Society of Breast Imaging. Eur Radiol 2008;18:1307-18.

4 6. Szumowski J, Coshow W, Li F, Coombs B, Quinn SF. Double-echo three-point- Dixon method for fat suppression MRI. Magn Reson Med 1995;34(1):120-4.

4 7. Sharma U, Danishad KK, Seenu V, Jagannathan NR. Longitudinal study of the assessment by MRI and diffusion-weighted imaging of tumor response in patients with locally advanced breast cancer undergoing neoadjuvant chemotherapy. NMR Biomed 2009;22:104-13.

4 8.Iacconi C, Giannelli M, Marini C, Cilotti A, Moretti M, Viacava P, et al. The role of mean diffusivity (MD) as a predictive index of the response to chemotherapy in locally advanced breast cancer: a preliminary study. Eur Radiol 2010;20:303-8.

49. Negendank W. Studies of human tumors by MRS: a review. NMR Biomed 1992;5(5):303-24.

50. Bartella L, Morris EA, Dershaw DD, Liberman L, Thakur SB, Moskowitz C, et al. Proton MR spectroscopy with choline peak as malignancy marker improves positive predictive value for breast cancer diagnosis: preliminary study. Radiology 2006;239(3):686-92.

51. Baek HM, Chen JH, Nalcioglu O, Su MY. Proton MR spectroscopy for monitoring early treatment response of breast cancer to neo-adjuvant chemotherapy. Ann Oncol 2008;19(5): 1022-4.

52. Kuhl CK, Mielcareck P, Klaschik S, Leutner C, Wardelmann E, Gieseke J, Schild HH. Dynamic breast MR imaging: are signal intensity time course data useful for differential diagnosis of enhancing lesions? Radiology. 1999 Apr;211(1):101-10.

53. Chopier J, Salem C, Billières P, Balleyguier C. Variation of the normal breast: mammographic and ultrasonographic aspects. Encycl Méd Chir 2003; 34-800-A-15.

54. Goumot PA, Bremond A, Dilhuydy MH, et al. La lecture mammographique : Sémiologie le sein normal. Le Sein : Son Image 1993.

55. Tabar L, Dean PB. Basic principals of mammogtaphic diagnosis. Diagn Imaging Clin Med 1985; 54 (3-4).

56. Meyer JE, Ferraro FA, Frenna TH, Di Piro PJ, Denison CM.

Mammographic appearance of normal intramammary lymph nodes in an atypical location. AJR Am J Roentgenol 1993; 161: 779-780.

57. Wolfe JN.Astudy of breast parenchyma by mammography in the normal woman and those with benign and malignant disease of the breast. Radiology 1967; 89: 210-215

58. Davros WJ, Madsen EL, Zagzebski JA. Breast mass detection by US: a phantom study. Radiology 1985; 156: 773-775.

59. D'Orsi CJ et al. ACR BI-RADS -Æ Atlas, Breast Imaging Reporting and Data System. Reston, VA, American College of Radiology; 2013.

60. Jokich PM, Monticciolo DL, Adler YT. Breast ultrasonography. Radiol Clin North Am 1992; 30: 993-1009.

61. Michelin J, Levy L. Normal breast and its variants: Diagnostic and interventional breast ultrasound. Collection d'imagerie radiologique. Masson, 1999; 9-13.

62. Neel-Paprocki V. Echo-anatomical reminders. Le Sein, 1994; 4: 73-77.

63. Garbay JR. Anatomy of the breast and axillary region. Breast Cancer Surgery: Diagnostic, Curative and Reconstructive 1997; 3-17.

64. Gallardo X, Sentis M, Castaner E, et al. Enhancement of intramammary lymph nodes with lymphoid hyperplasia: a potential pitfall in breast MRI. Eur Radiol. 1998;8: 1662-5.

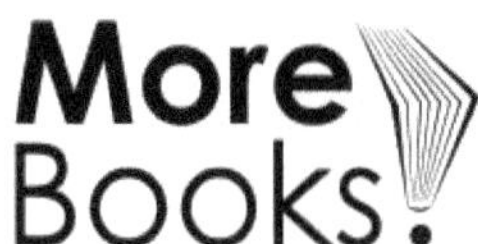

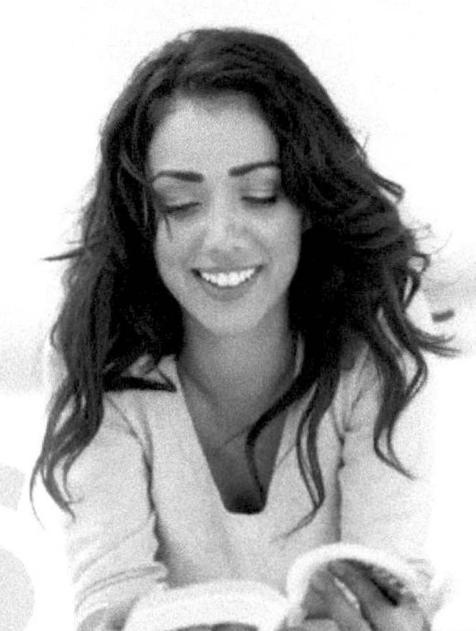

yes

I want morebooks!

Buy your books fast and straightforward online - at one of world's fastest growing online book stores! Environmentally sound due to Print-on-Demand technologies.

Buy your books online at
www.morebooks.shop

Kaufen Sie Ihre Bücher schnell und unkompliziert online – auf einer der am schnellsten wachsenden Buchhandelsplattformen weltweit! Dank Print-On-Demand umwelt- und ressourcenschonend produziert.

Bücher schneller online kaufen
www.morebooks.shop

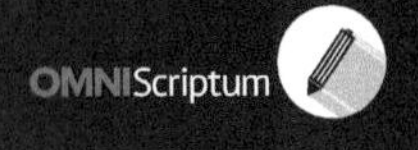

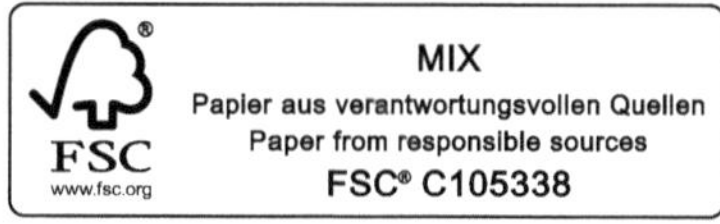

Printed by Books on Demand GmbH, Norderstedt / Germany